# YOUR HEALTH IS YOUR WEALTH

# YOUR HEALTH IS YOUR WEALTH

**PRINCE TOE SR.**

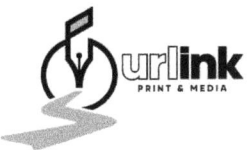

*Your Health is Your Wealth*

Copyright © 2019 by Prince Toe Sr. All rights reserved.

---

No part of this publication may be reproduced, stored in a retrieval system or transmitted in any way by any means, electronic, mechanical, photocopy, recording or otherwise without the prior permission of the author except as provided by USA copyright law.

The opinions expressed by the author are not necessarily those of URLink Print and Media.

---

1603 Capitol Ave., Suite 310 Cheyenne, Wyoming USA 82001
1-888-980-6523 | admin@urlinkpublishing.com

URLink Print and Media is committed to excellence in the publishing industry.

Book design copyright © 2019 by URLink Print and Media. All rights reserved.

---

Published in the United States of America
ISBN 978-1-64367-613-5 (Paperback)
ISBN 978-1-64367-612-8 (Digital)

27.06.19

# CONTENTS

1. Why did I choose this title? ................................. 7
2. Early Morning Prayers ...................................... 13
3. Morning Routine ............................................. 14
4. The Baby And The Stroller *(Cardio Workout)* ..... 16
5. Different Variation of Exercises and My Workout Routines ................................ 20
6. Drink lot of water ............................................ 23
7. Hard Work, Dedication, Consistency and Patience ....................................................... 25
8. Genetic Myth .................................................. 32
9. Sleep is Very Important .................................... 35
10. You Know Your Body Better Than Anybody Else ................................................. 37
11. Staying Natural Is Your Choice ......................... 39
12. Doing Steroids Is Your Choice ......................... 41
13. Adapt and Improvise ....................................... 43
14. Listen to Your Coaches ................................... 45
15. Eating Healthy ................................................ 48
16. Dieting ........................................................... 52
17. Competition ................................................... 55
18. Musclemania and Politics ................................ 57
19. The Networking .............................................. 60
20. Traveling ........................................................ 62
21. Fitness is a lifestyle ........................................ 64

# WHY DID I CHOOSE THIS TITLE?

Well, I chose this title for a lot of reasons. For the same reasons that will make anyone to read this book. This title is not just a title, but it is something for you to pay close attention as you are reading this book. This book is a self-help, powerful and unique way on his own. I am a strong believer when it comes to fitness and also when it comes to writing a fitness book. I precisely have to be very careful about how I chose my title. This is a book title that anyone and everybody can relate to. Your Health Is Your Wealth. What does the title really mean by that? First of all, when you think clearly, sit down at a quiet place and read the title again, you will realize that our health is everything. Our health is what we are. We are so focused on having materials wealth but seem to forget about the most precious in life that we have which is our health. It is not just only a title, but it's to remind everyone of us that our number one priority on this earth is taking care of our health and to stay healthy. With good health, you can achieve some things, but with better health, a person can achieve much more and the greatest things in life. Your Health Is Your Wealth when you really think about it. Why is that? Ask yourself those questions and as you read this book, you finally get to realize things that you taught were so important to you aren't and things that you long ago neglected are the most important things. Your health is life, and everything. Your Health Is Your Wealth is a title that makes anyone who reads my book wonder why I chose this title. I intentionally chose this title because of lot reasons: My personal experiences, Fitness, and others... For instance, there are certain things in life that money can't buy, neither helps you with, but a healthy lifestyle comes with those things that money cannot buy and give you. Living healthy is the best way of living and you destined to do so. Living Healthy comes with many good things in the long run. First one is that you don't have to worry about certain diseases either like the average person who constantly sees the doctors every other month. When you are healthy, happiness comes with it. One with a healthy lifestyle lives better, longer, happy and has better controlled over his/her life than the average person. Your Health Is Your Wealth is the book that everyone needs to read, wants to read and will want to read when It comes to getting in shape, motivation, staying in shape and even learn those different types of workouts, diet plan and use fitness as a lifestyle. In my book, I explain what I do in my daily life and morning routine etc. I also explain the different varieties of exercises I continuously do to stay in shape and fit. I also give examples, testimonies, and stories about my fitness life. This book is way different from any other fitness books you will read due to the facts, people who do fitness as a lifestyle, and especially me from my humble beginning was a struggle that I had to go through and now it's a journey that I am pursuing. Whosoever read this book, I want you to enjoy it and hope it gets to inspire you the way it inspires me every day to reach my fitness goals, to better myself and completely make fitness as part of my lifestyle. I am writing this book because I strongly feel that I hold this to myself and others who for years have been staying in shape, continuously staying shape and even making fitness to become part of their lives. I know it's not easy to reach those goals and hope for those who have just started but reading this book will change your mindset, doubts that you have had to exercise and taking your health seriously. Everything you want to know about my fitness lifestyle, it's all in this book. This is not only about fitness alone, but a book that will take you on a journey of a young man who perhaps fell in love with fitness. This book will completely change your life, show you how to stay focus and stay focus when you go to the gym.

My name is Prince B Toe Sr and I go by the nickname PRC MEMBER and also PRC. I was born in Liberia, Monrovia. I was raised by the late Makoula Odette who was my grandmother. I am the older child on my mother's side and the youngest on my father's side. My father passed away when my mother was pregnant with me. I never knew and neither met my father, I don't even know how he looks like and cannot imagined how will he looks like now if he was alive. Anyway, please don't feel sorry for me because I put behind my sorrows and moved forward. I was raised by the most beautiful, and loving woman Makoula Odette who taught me everything in my life and mostly the importance of life. I really don't know how Monrovia looks like and a little bit of knowledge that I have, it has been stuck in my memories forever.

My grandmother was a businesswoman, she and I, we both together traveled a lot during those years spent. For a woman, I had learned a lot and a lot of things from her that school won't teach. She was my father and mother at the same time. Even though as a child I had my moments of disobedience, Odette was always there to discipline and show me the right path. I know this book is about fitness, but it's mainly because of Makoula Odette I am where I am today. I hold my life to Odette. By 1989 and early 1990s, Most of the Liberians, Odette and I, we fled Liberia, Monrovia to move to the Ivory Coast because of the civil war which occurred. The Ivory Coast was one of the nearest neighbors' countries that Liberia shared a border with and was also the native country of Makoula Odette's who turned out to be my grandmother. Ivory Coast is a French-speaking country. Now as a child or a little boy you want to call it, I had to learn a whole new language and that was very hard for me. As I lived my life in the Ivory Coast, I became more familiar with their language, culture, lifestyle and mostly their macho attitude which I was mostly fascinated by the moment arrived. They took that lifestyle upon themselves. The Ivoirians were good people, but they have their macho and superheroes who I really admired when it came down to the fitness world. They were called Brigands and Bellards. Those are the two names that come into mind when I think about bodybuilding during the time spent in the Ivory Coast. I called them real bodybuilders with no steroids, but through their dedication, hard work and consistency that they achieve masterpiece that others are dying to have. They did it naturally and that alone it amazes me still now today date even though I'm abroad and have all the amenities that I need to transform my body. I wanted to be like them, they were like action heroes and wanted to be an action hero. I wanted to have an amazing physique like them and have a physique that no one can question. I wanted to be the one. I wanted to be strong, solid and powerful. Those Brigands and Bellards have created a physique every tourist admired and at the same time was afraid off due to the way they lived their lives. They were legends and Icons in their fields and loved by their people. Now let proceed to the next topic.

 # EARLY MORNING PRAYERS

I pray early in the morning before I go on by with my day. As a child, I was raised as Baptiste which I strongly arguably will say it is considered Christianity. Every morning when I wake up and every nighttime before I go to bed, I kneel down and say thank you to God almighty, beg for forgiveness and ask him to give me the strength to fight the unknown, bless my family and watch over us as we close our eyes for bedtime. Thank him for what is already mine and keep on blessing me and my family so we can bless others in need. I strongly believe that the man upstairs is the one who is making it possible for me and keep blessing me with gifts that others will die for to have. Prayers in my life are very important and play important roles in my daily life. Through prayers and exercising that's how I fight my demons, stay humble, calm, stay patient regardless of the outcomes. It's like meditating, but spiritually and physically at the same time and all that combine in one. After praying, now I can do my Morning Routine.

 # MORNING ROUTINE

I will set my timer on my smartphone for 30 minutes for me to stretch my muscles and the whole entire body. First thing I do the head touch the knees while standing up. It's one of my favorite exercises I do from time to time. What it does to your body that, it creates that flexibility. Even though it's uncomfortable, but as you practice for a long period of time, it starts to get easy and enjoyable. First, you have your legs straight and make sure your knees aren't bending for you to feel the maximum stretch when your head is touching your knees. As you do so, breathing also plays an important part in this. Inhale as you straighten your legs and knees and while your head is going to touch your knees exhale to feel the maximum burn in the muscles and so of the whole body. This exercise also helps loosening your hamstrings, lower back muscles and even also helps prevent back injuries due to stiff or tight hamstrings. I do that for 5 minutes the most and I switch to another stretching exercise. The second exercise I love to do it's the Vandame's splits. I love doing splits because Vandamme is my idol and I look up to him and he is the first reason as I child I started exercising. Anyway, enough with the splits, the first thing I do, I wear both of my socks, and slowly do the splits all the way down and stay down for another 5 minutes. Feel the intense and painful burn in my legs and my muscles. It hurts so bad that it makes you want to quit, but don't because pain doesn't kill. Pain is temporary. She either lasts for a moment, day, weeks, months, years and even longtime, but she is not here to stay, my friend. After I am done stretching, I fix myself a healthy breakfast. I usually fix myself an omelet, oatmeal and a glass of concentrated fresh orange juice and two slices of wheat bread or sometimes bagels. After I am done eating my breakfast, I relax for about 15 to 20 minutes for the food to digest. After that, it's show time. My next routine is a special one and it is called Baby and The Stroller. Most of the times when people or a person hears me talking about the Baby and the Stroller; one will automatically think and strictly assumes that it is a mother and her child. Perhaps I guess they are wrong on this one because this is a father and son duo workout.

# THE BABY AND THE STROLLER
## (CARDIO WORKOUT)

The Baby And The Stroller is the name that I came up with. Since I am a father of four and my last born is only two years old and spends time with me before work. When I go run, I will take him with me in the stroller. I realize that he loves to workout also and enjoy the run. The Baby and the Stroller has saved my life in a way that I'm so grateful. Before my son Gabriel was born, I was working out early after I dropped the rest two of children to school and my wife dropped off the third child to her school. Since Gabriel was born, things have changed gradually for every one of us in the house and especially me. My workout routines have also changed and it was irritating and frustrating for me because I take my workout routines very seriously. Eventually, a great idea comes along which is using the baby stroller while I go run with my little man. The first day was a little bit awkward, but still, winners always find ways to progress and turn uncomfortable situations to comfortable. This is a father and son duo workout routine that is a just little different from the rest, but they are doing what they love to do. I put the baby in the baby stroller, keep him comfy with a blanket, jacket on him, baby bottle in his stroller's pocket and pacifier in his mouth and it's time to go. We both excited, but no words are said to one another, perhaps only glance from eye contact we both know it is going to be an amazing ride and as more to come. I have all the tools I needed. The baby and I, we are both ready for this run with his pieced blue eyes which look likes his mom are intentionally looking at me and thinking I am one of the super dads who is really cool. A smile on my face and inside I'm screaming out loud saying: "Yes I am really cool, little crazy and so of you. You are your old man and part of me also. You will be a legend just like me hahahaha." The stroller, the baby and I, three of us are ready to do the impossible. Both hands are on the handles of the stroller as tight as they can be Batman and Robin are warming up, things are about to get real, the future legend and Icon are getting ready for that iconic run. Suddenly, the slow walks began to fasten, the pace is picking up, now my baby boy is getting excited because he knows how this long ride goes and adventurous it is. First, we are going up the hill which usually is a warm up before we go to war. Like father, like son and this is the lifestyle we both choose especially me and since at a younger age. We are still going up the hill and it is not an easy thing to do at all, but this what I choose to do rest of my life till the breath of life vanishes from my lungs. The pain is not that bad at all, but the burns and my lower back is telling me to give up. Still, I'm moving forward, my breathing is getting thicker, but before I used to gasp for air. I guess my body starts to adjust to this cruel workout that lots of athletes are escaping, but here I am doing with my son in his stroller. We are moving on the sidewalk as if I was a machine on wheels. The only thing that is following as swiftly as me it's my shadow.

Still, I feel the burns in my legs also but I can't give up now, I have come too far to be giving up. The struggle and pain are real. I can't make this stuff up at all. Pain is just temporary, but quitting is for life and I am one of those human beings that never quits until I see results. Voice in my head is my motivation right now. My son is, on the other hand, dying with excitement, but he still a baby and learning how to talk. From his body language and the way he calls my name, I absolutely know he is excited. Finally, we have gotten to the peak of the hill, I finally realize how far I have come and accomplished in this fitness world and also my daily life. Two years ago, I barely run 2 miles without struggling; now it seems like a walk to the park. My body is finally adapting to the abuse I put her through in the past several years. My body is finally starting to understand the fundamentals of this workout. I need this workout to show the world how crazy my physique and with the proper technique of workout, it can be done. Enough talking, let get back to business, now we have to run back from where we started and here we go. I am in the zone and in my own world where no one can stop me and focus on the bigger price. I stand tall, my legs are on the verge of giving up, but it's all mental now from now on. I feel the pain and agonies but I am who I am. I love doing this and this is what makes me different from others. We are repeating the same cycle, but going back. I'm out of breath and mentally I am there and will finish this run. Legs are sored, I'm thirsty and those two bottles of water I brought with me, one is gone already. However, I can drink too much water because I need the water to finish my run. As I began with my run going back, one thing that comes into mind its win,

win and win. Telling myself suffer now, go through the pain now and reap the fruits of your labor later. I'm back in the zone. How we are going to win if I can't adapt with the uncomfortable asking myself this question over and over. This is the life I choose. This is the route that I decided to take on and follow it regardless of the outcomes. As I breathe in again, suddenly I began to absorb the fresh given air from the man's upstairs. The fresh air started to help my lungs to recover from the fatigue and my body starts to understand why this gruesome workout that I'm putting her through. Hopefully one day, she understands the love that I'm giving her and how beautiful I want her to look among others. I want her to look as good out of clothes and in clothes as always. My mind is getting back to her normal state again. Here we go again, running on the sidewalk, sweat dripping off my body, hungry for more and all I am thinking about it's the phenomenal physique that I am trying to create. A sight to see, something that no one has ever seen in the whole entire life before and to me, my body is an artwork and just began to understand her.

    I can do whatever I want to do to her, but she has to understand the fundamentals of my craziness first and we can proceed with our plan. As we are making it back, I began to realize that my fatigue completely does this thing called Endorphins and are been produced in our bodies. I have refreshed again and seemed I just began running. Instead of two miles a day on my days off, now I began to run ten miles to twenty miles when I combined both days.

# DIFFERENT VARIATION OF EXERCISES AND MY WORKOUT ROUTINES

Since it is Monday, the first day of the week, I only do body workout which means I don't use any weight at all. I will set my timer on my cell phone for an hour and a half and then, I will choose a workout. For example, I choose to do pushups but in different varieties and also choose a number of pushups I'm going to do. For example, I will choose 1000 pushups which I will divide it into 4 sections and each variation of pushups I will be doing will be 250 each. My first section of pushups will be Incline Pushups which are my favorites because of lots of reasons. Incline Pushups is a unique and complete exercise. When a person is doing incline pushups, a person is also working on the chest, triceps, shoulders and also back muscles. A person also works on the lower chest and more on back. There are several benefits of doing incline pushups. For instance, incline pushups is a relatively simple bodyweight exercise that primarily works the pectoral muscles in addition to the sternal component of the pectoralis major. Incline Pushups also target the clavicular pectoralis, triceps, and biceps. After when I'm done doing the incline pushups, I will switch the Decline Pushups which most likely called Regular Pushups if I'm not mistaking. Decline Pushups which are also called Regular Pushups are designed to work mostly on the upper chest and front shoulders (Delts). Decline Pushups or Regular Pushups help tremendously for a fitter and mainly focus on your arms, abs, and lower body. They also educate or train muscles to work together and become stronger. Decline Pushups or Regular Pushups help to create balance and stability according to David Nordmark, author of the book Pushups for Everyone: Perfect Pushups Workout for Muscle Growth, Strength and Endurance (Home Workout Routines, build muscle, strength training, exercise workout Book3). Decline Pushups or Regular Pushups help you get a stronger midsection and upper body. It incorporates the stabilization muscles of your core, combining an upper body pushing movement with a plan. It also is in fact that one of the best and most basic exercises of the midsections. After when I'm done with this variation of pushups, I begin with my different variation abs workouts. I strongly believe that different abs workout makes your abs chiseled. My first abs workout its crunches and perhaps I assume everyone knows what I'm talking about. I hate them what I'm doing them but love them after I'm done doing them because they make my abs look great. They make my abdominal section look amazing. Anyone can do crunches, but there's a proper way of doing them. First, you lay on the floor with both knees bent and both feet flat on the ground. I will say approximately about a foot from your lower back and place your fingertips on your temple with your palms facing out. When you are done doing so, you draw your belly into the base of your spine to engage the muscles, and then raise your head and shoulders off the floor. Repeat the whole thing again as much as you want and feel like it. Second Abs Workout it is called laying legs raises with ankles weights on. First you start off laying on your back on the floor with your arms palms down on either side, keep your legs together and as straight as possible as you can and slowly raise your legs to a 90-degree angle, pause for few seconds at this position as high as you can reach your legs, and then slowly lower your legs back down while your abdominal muscle contraction. If it is too hard for you to do, please safety comes first. Remove the ankle weights and do it without the ankle weights. As for me, I'm used to doing with the ankle weights due to the years of experience and training. And my last abs workout is called plank and it is one of my favorite workouts. Forearm Plank, first you place your forearms on the ground with your elbows bent at a 90-degree angle aligned beneath your shoulders with your arms parallel at your shoulders width. Second, your feet should be together with only your toes should be touching the floor and lift your belly off the floor and form a straight line from your heels to the crown of your head, then hold tightly as much you can.

# DRINK LOT OF WATER

Drinking Lot of Water during Workout and Daily, most of us and especially athletes, we do know the importance of water already but still due to our stubbornness and negligence that we do not intake the amount of water that needed to be taking. When the water level of our plasma is high, less water is reabsorbed into the blood and our urine is more dilute when we exercise, we get hot, increase sweating and lose a lot of water and perhaps the blood plasma becomes more concentrated. This is where drinking water plays a very important part in our bodies. Water is necessary for our body. Water replaces those lost sweats that came out of our body during exercising. It's a must for your body because water regulates your body temperature and helps lubricate your joints. Water also helps transport nutrients to give you energy and perhaps keep you healthy. Without enough water into your body, your body can't perform at her best. For instance, bodybuilder like me has to drink a lot of water because of several reasons. Water and Bodybuilding have something in common. Drink water help to build muscles and get shredded. Drinking enough water helps you build muscle and perhaps lose fat also more efficiently because your body is functioning optimally on a cellular level. Drinking a lot of water is also cleansing your body and proper hydration is the key of dieting in bodybuilding. It also goes to the average person who doesn't work out; he/she still has to drink water because drinking is very important for every one of us. An average person has to drink 8 ounces glass of water a day and that's considered healthy. Perhaps if you want to stay dehydrated please make sure you drink up to 8 ounces glass of water every day too. However, it might change depending on how much the person weight and size also. If a person weights more and bigger than the average person, the person might consume more water. For people to stay hydrated, make sure you drink your 8 ounces of water each day. Your body is made of 50-65 percent of water while the ideal range for women is between 45 and 60 percent study shows. Studies also show that in adult men, about 60 percent of their bodies are water. However, fat tissue does not have as much water as lean tissue and in adult women; fat makes up more the body than men. They have 55 percent of their bodies made of water. Perhaps I recommend People should follow those guidelines that are in my book to stay hydrated and now I will proceed to the next interesting topics of my next chapter.

# HARD WORK, DEDICATION, CONSISTENCY AND PATIENCE

Those are the rules that I follow in my daily life. There is no magic, shortcuts, and miracles if you want to be successful especially in the bodybuilding world. Hard Work, Dedication, Consistency and Patience are the four main ingredients that a person needs to make in the bodybuilding world, other avenues one may choose to take and in life general. Without those four things, you won't make it. We all have dreams, want to be a star, famous, popular and great, but if you don't put actions behind your dreams, your dreams become an empty promise in the wind. For those dreams to become reality, you must decide and make difficult decisions and put yourself in an uncomfortable position where you only think about are your dreams and how you are going to make them come true. After putting yourself in the uncomfortable position and tell yourself you are going to make it regardless of the outcomes which lead to Hard Work. When it comes to Hard Work, everyone is entitled of their own opinion and has their own definition of Hard Work. I'm not the strongest, but I work hard when it comes to my dreams. I always tell myself that a closed mouth doesn't get fed. I love beautiful things and to have those things in my life, I will work hard to get them.

Now I am in the position to make my dreams come true and God Bless America! If have to wake up 2 or 3 am in the morning to make sure that everything is in order for my dreams; I won't hesitate at all to do that. I strongly believe that the harder you work, the easy it gets. I also believe that Hard Work is there to pave the way for success. Hard Work is the key to success also and paves the easy chemin ahead for us for the future. For example, I'm a father of four, wife, work full time, and go to school part-time and workout twice a day. Others might say that I'm crazy; they are the ones who are not me. My vision is cleared and I can see it clearly. Those are my dreams and not theirs. Those are my dreams and will work on them as hard as anyone else. I'm the chauffeur of my vehicle and I have to set examples for myself. I have dreams and I will accomplish them before I leave this earth. My mindset is arguably my strongest friend right at this moment. If have to work thousand times harder than everyone else. If have to walk 100 miles a day to get my dreams and make them come true, I will do it in a blink of an eye. If it causes to sleep in my car to be where I need and want to be I will do it without hesitation. I'm not holding anything back or giving up on my dreams. I will keep trying until I see results or collapse while trying. Hard Work is the key to success, but without Dedication, it is a waste of time, effortless because Dedication is everything and has to do it with everything.

    Dedication is very important to dreamers, business people and anyone who is trying to do something special in this world. If you are not dedicated to your craft, you won't make it and that's the naked truth, my friend. You have to breathe, eat and sleep with dedication on your mind as always. You hold it to yourself. Hard work alone won't solve the puzzle and the problems with your goals. You have to be full time committed. One has to devote their time to his task and complete to see positive outcomes. You have to ask yourself if is that you really want to do? Dedication is easy to say it, but most of us can't even devote our times in to dream, but can devote our times into making others people dreams come true. Dedication is like a marriage. You have to be faithful when things are going great and when things aren't going so great. All I'm trying to say that, sometimes you feel like you don't want to do anything, Bang bang bang! Wake up! This is the time where you have to discipline your mind because when you are tired and feeling lazy, this is where you give your all and the best comes out of you. You have to be mentally prepared for whatever it takes for you to make your dreams come to reality and that's the truth. You have to be stubborn, violent and even aggressive toward them and let them know you are the fire in the making. You have to sacrifice, cut off bad habits, stay focus and passionate about your dreams, even some days are going to be your lowest point, but still, find a way to work on them and keep on dreaming. Those are your dreams and they are your battles. You have to fight for them to bring them alive. You have to punish yourself and worked as hard more than anyone else on your craft every day so you can master it. Dedication is when you are so tired and don't want to do anything, but still proceed to work on your dreams anyway. It's when you are supposed to go out on the weekend with friends, but refuse to go and choose to stay at home to work on your dreams. You need to have a purpose to see the big picture, be a visionary and have the drive that everyone doesn't have but only you. You need to have that hunger inside that wants more and that fire that won't stop burning. After you master and learn how to be dedicated, perhaps you also need to add Consistency to your bucket list.

What is Consistency" It means something staying the same. It also means that you have to keep working every second, every minute, every hour, every day, every week, every month, and every year on the same dreams until you see results on the project. This is how you get better at something. You have to discipline yourself mentally and keep on working on your craft over and over to finish the task you plan to do. For example, to have the consistency of what you do, one must create a specific goal or goals that you want to accomplish in a short term and long term. One must create a schedule or a planner that will help place reminder around your home, workplace etc. Make a promise that you can keep and give yourself something every time you finish the task. Your consistency has to be very polished. What I mean by that is that you have to beat on your craft every day until you can't any longer. For instance, in the bodybuilding world, one of the famous words is No Pain No Gain. It means that if you don't lift heavy you won't be big and that's the same mentality you should have toward your goals. Keep knocking at the door until someone finally comes to open the door. This is how you should with your craft because once you master it, everything else comes easy. At the end of the day, it comes to one thing to accomplish which are your dreams and its one the most difficult thing that lot of us are having the problem with and still now. Hard Work, Dedication and Consistency do play a major role in your dreams, but the most important is Patience because it's the virtue of all.

Patience is everything. You will need one if you want to be successful because it's very important and powerful. Patience is a virtue to all. Patience is the final recipe. As a human being and when I was a child, I had an anger problem, but as I get older, I realize that to become successful at anything will require patience and that's the naked truth. This goes with everything I do in my daily life and especially in the bodybuilding. It has been 20 years since I been working out, but approximately 4 years since I have been doing bodybuilding. As I grow into the bodybuilding world, I realize that I'm still a student to this game. Things that I thought I knew were just the tip of the iceberg. Bodybuilding is an art, not just a sport and different kind of breed of sport. I realize that it takes more than just Hard Work, Dedication and Consistency. Patience summarizes all of them. As I get deeper in the bodybuilding world, participate in events, compete and experience other avenues of it. Patience is the capacity to accept or tolerate delay, trouble or suffering without getting angry or upset. For me as a bodybuilder, sometimes I expect certain body parts to be equal as others and to look better as the others, but it doesn't always work like that. Anything that is good takes time and even greater will need more time. From my four years doing bodybuilding, I had learned one of the most valuable things which are called Patience. Before I had any clue and was frustrated from time to time. For a while, I was depressed and was too harsh on myself, but I still smile. I frequently act like everything was good, but inside I wanted fast results and demanded some answers why I'm not where I want to be... Why it is taking too long? I asked my cousin Grady who introduces me to this bodybuilding world and also one of my coaches. He laughed and said to me, "Pekin you have to be patient." That is the naked truth. It takes time. As days have gone by, weeks have gone by, months have gone by and years have gone by, I began to see a transformation take place from my hard work, dedication, and consistency. I began to see the symmetry in my legs, my weak abs muscles which start to turn solid and the majority of my body parts began to transform also. From that moment I realize, being Patience, it is everything in life. Sometimes in life, we want something so bad that we will do anything in our power to get there, but we lack the most important ingredient which is called Patience. Lack of Patience becomes our downfall in life period. We work hard; dedicate our lives to our crafts and not forgetting about consistency. One thing that most of us don't have including me is Patience. We intend to somehow forget or I will call it not having faith in ourselves and our crafts. We let all those three things to go into waste and everything in vain. I will tell you this story that I got from listening to Les Brown who is my favorite motivational speaker about the Chinese Bamboo Tree and how long it takes for the Bamboo Tree to grow. It is said that the Chinese Bamboo Tree begins as a nut, a hard nut about the size of a walnut, but in the fifth year, the Chinese Bamboo Tree finally breaks through the ground and this is how your patience should be. Not because you are not seeing the results physically, it doesn't mean that they are not there. They are just not in season yet that's why. The next topic that I'm about to talk about is the Genetic Myth which plays a huge part in the Bodybuilding world.

 # GENETIC MYTH

Genetic Myth is a huge issue in the Bodybuilding community and still, I don't understand why. People are so concerned and can't wait to categorize others physiques instead of worrying about themselves. I think it is a weakness when another person focuses on another person genetics. It is something that makes me laugh every time whenever I hear them saying that. I am not an expert in human genetics, but I strongly feel that it just an excuse for people to not give their all and 100% in the gym when he/she is working out. I strongly disagree with the Genetic Theory because we are all created equal and we are all gifted when it comes to anything and especially Bodybuilding. In my opinion, I strongly believe that the Genetic Myth Conspiracy that is going on, it's all mental and I will tell you why I think this way. From the beginning of time, especially in America, every human being believes that black people are very superiors when it comes to entertainment: sport, music etc. That alone that is the advantage that we black people will and forever have over any other race. Even if we were not are not gifted, but the world alone has given us more confidence and we feel like we have no choice but to be great. It is like a law of attraction. Whatever you think, will come to the past because if you feel you are the greatest bodybuilder, eventually you will become or be very soon. Another example, society perhaps believes that Asian people are very smart and intelligent. I will disagree with that. I'm not taking anything from them either and I respect them very much. I strongly believe they are hardworking people who want a great future and they work hard for what they have. As for the Genetic Myth, I think it's all in the mind and a lot of people are falling for it. Another example, if you look up the definition of White, you will notice that the meaning will tell you that everything that has to do with White is pure, good and angelic, but the definition of Black is evil, bad and demonic. So, from that alone, it's a lesson that we all need to learn from and not let others' assumptions to affect our greatness and that goes with the same with the Genetic Myth. If you work at something, eventually great results will show. Like my cousin Grady said to me when people tell him he looks great, he looks this way because of his genetic at the end of their speeches, Grady replies by being sarcastic "what happened to yours in a funny way?" By the way, which I really find very funny, I strongly believe we are all created equal including men and women. Whatever your mind thinks, you can achieve and Grady is a great example. During the past years, I watched this young man turned to a great bodybuilder because he loves his craft and he works very hard every day on his craft. The whole Genetic Myth is a placebo. It's for lazy people and those are who always making up excuses to not go to the gym or try to better themselves. It is also for jealous people who can't accomplish what others accomplish but instead using the race card as a lame excuse to make themselves feel good. The whole Genetic Myth thing is all in the mind. Like Bruce Lee said, "If you put the water in the cup, the water becomes the cup." So for the other race of people out there, there is nothing in this world that is impossible. Anything is achievable, but you need to get your mindset right to stay focus to achieve your goals. Water is shapeless and so of the Genetic Myth. I've seen several of white, Asian, and different race of bodybuilders who look better than the black bodybuilders. They work very hard to achieve their goals. It takes Hard work, Dedication, Consistency, and Patience to be on top and that goes to everyone. As I explain and give my opinion on the Genetic Myth, the next topic that I will talk about is the importance of sleep.

# SLEEP IS VERY IMPORTANT

The Importance of Sleep is a crucial problem that we as bodybuilders have and still have. It is affecting us all in whole as bodybuilders. We don't sleep or rest whatever you want to call it. We don't let our bodies to fully recharge. Everyone wants to be a beast and overwork our bodies without enough rest and sleep including me. I took me years and years for me to realize all my Hard work was not displaying as well I wanted it to. I am always tired due to lack of sleep and rest. Even though I work out five days a week and even sometimes six days a week, still I couldn't see great results, but stay exhausted every day. My soul mate will tell me that I needed to rest and get enough sleep so my body can recover. I wouldn't listen to her even though I knew she was right. I will still continue calling myself a beast because I see everyone doing it. I was strong. After I saw my size was getting smaller and that got my attention and makes me wonder what was going on with my body. Eventually, I realize that I need to sleep more and more rest so I can see any growth. In other for any muscle growth, you have to rest and sleep for the muscles to repair. How long does it take for a muscle to repair after a workout? Eccentric contractions cause more muscle damage and thus entail longer recovery. John Berardi, Ph.D., says "that taking everything into account, a given muscle will not fully recover until seven to 14 days have elapsed after a hard workout. However, you can resume your workouts after 48 hours of rest." Some research suggests that because muscle soreness can peak two days post-exercise, a minimum of 48 hours of rest is optimal to allow recovery and prevent injury—at least among the competitive athletes who were studied. If you want to see muscle growth, you have to follow those things that I listed. This is how you see results which lead to great as you do it often. Another thing that I also go to for a faster after an intense workout, I intend to sleep more, eat more foods that contain proteins, drink lot more of water and watch my couple of good action flicks which turn to my resting. As you can see, it takes those things to see changes in your body, so our next topic will be you have to know your body better than anyone else.

# YOU KNOW YOUR BODY BETTER THAN ANYBODY ELSE

A study shows that "Almost 99% of the mass of the human body is made up of six elements: oxygen, carbon, hydrogen, nitrogen, calcium, and phosphorus. Only about 0.85% is composed of another five elements: potassium, sulfur, sodium, chlorine, and magnesium." You Know Your Body Better Than Anybody Else is the key point to the whole fitness thing. You have to know what your body can and can't do at all times. I'm not trying to judge, but the majority of the people don't even know their own bodies that very well and will do anything to destroy her without even knowing. The body is a piece of art and believe it or not, but it is the naked truth. You have to find a niche for her. You have to do a workout that works for her and leave the ones that don't. Knowing your body better than anyone else can save you from a lot of injuries. The human skeleton is the internal framework of the body. It is composed of around 270 bones at birth – this total decreases to around 206 bones by adulthood after some bones get fused together and the bone mass in the skeleton reaches maximum density around age 21. The human skeleton of an adult consists of 206-208 bones. It is composed of 270 bones at birth but later decreases to 80 bones in the axial skeleton and 126 bones in the appendicular skeleton. You have to know all those things before you go at the head and start to do things that will cause you to regret in the long run. At least you have to know some of your muscles groups that are stronger than others by what exercise you see yourself doing often. You have to know your strengths and weaknesses before you let anyone train you or start giving you those crazy ideas. For example, whenever I'm at the gym I will see a person will pick up a weight that is three times their size and heavy than he can lift, but still trying to lift and I wonder why. I just don't look surprised anymore, but that smile on my face even though I know it is wrong but ego and pride that is what gets a person hurt in the gym. The mind might think otherwise, but the body thinks another way. So for he/she who tries to lift heavy, your mind and body have to connect first. They both have to agree upon the weights you are trying to lift. It might sound crazy to you, but you have to learn how to communicate with your body and perhaps your mind will also connect. As a bodybuilder and athlete, it has taken many years to figurate this, but it takes times to understand the whole philosophy behind it. Since then, it has helped me increase my weights and build my confidence every time I'm at the gym. He/she has to be careful when it comes to lifting and working out because one doesn't want him/her a lifetime injury. All I'm trying to say is that listen to your body very careful will prevent injuries, workout smart and not letting your ego get the best of you.

# STAYING NATURAL IS YOUR CHOICE

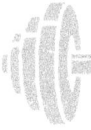

Staying Natural Is Your Choice and I, my friend I had made that choice a long time ago at the age of 16. Now that I'm 36 years of age and I look better than ever. I look great; feel great and also very happy. Staying Natural is part of my integrity and loyalty to those who workout and exercise naturally and burst their butts to create a decent physique. The whole Staying Natural is something that I believe in, it is sexy, and even give hope to others believing that they can achieve a decent physique also. Staying Natural is something that I truly believe in if you are doing fitness because you want to be fit and stay healthy. So for me as a natural bodybuilder, it is a challenge and I love the challenges of Staying Natural. I love challenges in my life and it is one of those that I enjoy doing. There is something unique about being a Natural Bodybuilder and Staying Natural. It puts you in a place that is vulnerable and makes you feel good about yourself because of the achievement you have accomplished. One thing I have to say about Staying Natural is that the things I went through with my transformation. If I tell you it's not hard, I am telling lies. It's hard to be a natural bodybuilder because of what you have to go through and also because of the duration of muscles growth.

So before you choose to be a Natural Bodybuilder or Staying Natural, rethink on your decisions because the route you are taking its far different from the others. What is a Natural Bodybuilder anyway? It is a bodybuilding movement with various competitors that take place for bodybuilders who abstain from performance-enhancing drugs. This categorically excludes the used of substances like anabolic steroids insulin, diuretics and human growth hormones. Being a Natural Bodybuilder means that you are not using, neither taking any supplement to help you for muscle growth and you are doing the natural way through your hard work. There are advantages to Staying Natural and being a Natural Bodybuilder. Being a Natural Bodybuilder and Staying Natural increases your lifespan. You live a healthy lifestyle and be proud of yourself in the humblest way that you are a living proof because of the world we are living in now where everything is taking over by supplements when it comes to fitness. You have worked hard to achieve a decent physique that a natural person can and will be able to achieve without any help of Steroids. The disadvantages of Staying Natural and being a Natural Body bodybuilder are Steroids.

# DOING STEROIDS IS YOUR CHOICE

Steroids, Steroids, Steroids, and Steroids are calling people and killing people. Before Steroids, we were all once natural and perhaps I will say we all started as natural. I guess things have changed as the world changes and the sport of bodybuilding becomes more demanding and not only that, everyone wants a quick fixed to look like what they have in mind. I have nothing against those who used it, but it is one thing that really bothers me. First thing is that those who claim to be natural, but damn well know that they are not and it bothers to the extent that I feel discussing. Why guys that on Steroids claim to be Natty which means Natural by the way. I still don't understand. It is something that I can't explain either will ever understand why they are claiming to do so. Is it because they missed being Natural or just saying that to erase the guilt? I don't know and I cannot tell you why they do that, but one thing I can tell you for sure it's that using Steroids is a choice and perhaps it just like everything else in life. I'm not interested in it. I am not an expert when it comes to Steroids, but the little that I know I will knowledge you on it. What is Steroids? Anabolic Steroid Use in Bodybuilding and Weightlifting, Anabolic agents are potent promoters of protein synthesis and thus are muscle building. Anabolic Steroids are usually androgenic, meaning that they enhance male characteristics—body hair, muscle, male genitalia, and deep voice. This is the definition of the use of Anabolic steroids. Some bodybuilders use drugs such as anabolic steroids and precursor substances such as prohormones to increase muscle hypertrophy. Other performance-enhancing substances used by competitive bodybuilders include human growth hormone (HGH), which can cause acromegaly. For those athletes and bodybuilders who claim to be natural, this what natural bodybuilders see on you when you are claiming that you are one of us. We see things that you don't see or ignoring to see. For example, several acne, frequent heart attack, rashes, oily skin, hair loss, liver diseases, such as liver tumors and cysts. Kidney disease, heart disease, such as heart attack and stroke, altered mood, irritability, increased aggression, depression or suicidal tendencies. Those are the things we see so please stop claiming that you are Natural because it is a disgrace for the Natural. I am not taking anything away from those who are using Steroids because no matter what, they still have to put in work to get where they are today with aid from Steroids. The next topic will be on Adapt and Improvise

 # ADAPT AND IMPROVISE

Adapt and Improvise is something that I love to do all the times especially when it comes to working out. I hear people saying I need a gym to workout. I need a gym to get in shape and to me its pure nonsense. You don't really need a gym to really workout and stay fit. If you really want to get in shape, you will look for ways to get in shape. If it is that important to you, you look for ideas and even create ideas to get in shape. For example, you can go to the park, run a couple laps around the soccer field, do a couple of pushups and sit-ups. You can even do pull-ups if the park has some pullups bars or can use the soccer poles bars. Another thing that you can do, it's that you can start doing lunges by using your body weight. You can also use the resistance bands to exercise with. They are a lot of things that you can do without going to the gym. Majority of the times, it's all in our head and believes that if we don't go to the gym, we can't get in shape. Adapt and Improvise is always in my head because when I travel to a location where there are any gym and any weight, I use to Adapt and Improvise to my own advantage. For example, some hotels don't have any gym, so what I do? I use my own body weight to work out or exercise. I will do jumping jacks, use water bottles for curls and especially the 16oz for triceps workout and use the chair or couch in my hotel room to do some shoulders workout. Sometimes I even use my better half to sit on my back while I do some prison pushups and use the wall to do standing squat. There is always something to do if you open your mind and let your mind work and believe me when I say it, you will have so many great ideas that she generates when it comes to workout without needing the gym. This is going to all bodybuilders and athletes, I know it's not enough for us, but use this great idea to maintain your physique for now till you get to a location where they have gym's equipment. Adapt and Improvise my friend and use that any part of the world where you go. The next topic will be Listen To Your Coaches.

# LISTEN TO YOUR COACHES

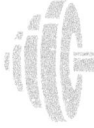

Listen to Your Coaches is very important to all athletes and especially Bodybuilders like me. I have learned my lesson a few years ago when I went to South Miami Beach to compete at Musclemania. A few years back I went to South Miami Beach to compete, I was ready and felt that I was on top of the world. While there I was supposed to do my tan, but I refused to do so after Mama Ruby who is a mentor and my other mother now as we speak today told me to do tan; but I refused to do so for being cheap and no listening. I had learned my lesson that weekend by not winning anything at all and placing at all. Listening to your coaches will really do you a huge favor, but perhaps also you have to be careful and watch out for those who called themselves Fitness Gurus. They are many of them out there portraying to be Fitness experts, but they have any clue about Fitness. They have the true Fitness gurus out there and when you see them you will automatically know what I'm talking about. They know exactly what they are talking about and doing. As for me I was really lucky and blessed to have a great team, experts and know about Fitness. They are also my mentors when it comes to fitness. They have carried me underneath their wings and taught me everything I know about

Bodybuilding, fitness; show the secrets and tricks about the whole fitness game. Now let's start from the beginning my fitness journey, I was just a normal average person who and a guy who loves to work out and mostly focus on the upper body, lifting heavy, mostly trying to get bigger and was also neglecting my others body parts. I started doing Bodybuilding 4 years ago and Grady Gray the Co-Founder of the GrayAtlas apparels took me underneath his wings and taught me lots of things about Bodybuilding and Fitness that I had any clue. Bodybuilding and Fitness are not about working out, but it's an art. You have to understand the body and the workouts that she needs and each body part also needs. Even though I am older than Grady, but this kid has taught me a lot about Bodybuilding and Fitness. Not a day, I will let my pride takes over. I always listen to him because I know he knows a lot and knows exactly what he is talking about and doing. In this sport of Bodybuilding and Fitness, I am still looking at myself as a student of this sport and that's how a Wiseman learns. Grady has taught me and a lot and introduced me to his whole team since he lives overseas. Through Grady, I met Osei Bonsu his business partner, the co-founder of GrayAtlas who always been there for me since day one. Took me in as a brother and taught me more tricks about fitness, what to do and not do. I also met brother Duke, Raquel, the whole team California and especially Mama Ruby who is everybody mom and also my mentor. Since I met those great people, my whole fitness life has changed so of my physique. Been around those beautiful people have also motivated me more and give me the strength to work harder because they are in top shape and inspired me to be at my best. They have my best interest; want me to be at my best and see me successful. Only a few people in this world can do that for you. Meeting mama Ruby and getting to know her more reminds me of lots about my grandmother who raised me. Mama Ruby is a living legend, a living proof in the Fitness World and in life period. Mama Ruby has taken me under her wings, coach me about life and so many things that I needed to know and hear about the fitness industry and the process you have to go through. She has taken me in as her own son and will always be real from day one since I met her through my cousin Grady. Because of that, I got more attached to her and even gain more respect for her and for being truly a mentor who doesn't only want to see me winning a championship but do great in life because she believes in me. She believes in me so much that sometimes I feel so special hahhahaha. Even during workout section with Mama Ruby, It is a learning process because every day there is something new that I learn from the Queen Of Fitness which it is the name I gave her by the way. For her age, you will think she will slow down, but you are wrong because every day during the workout section, I get amazed by her. Workouts she does and shows me are very hard and work, but also very effective. Even though I have a few years in Bodybuilding now, but I still consider myself a student to this sport. There are lots more I need to learn and I'm waiting to explore. As the story goes on, the next topic talks about Eating Healthy.

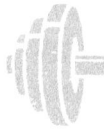 # EATING HEALTHY

Eating Healthy is very important to the average person, athletes and mostly Bodybuilders. I was far from and that's the truth. I will only eat healthy when there is an upcoming show that I have to do. I was not disciplined at all. I was almost eating everything as foods wise. Mostly I was eating greasy, oily and fast foods majority of the times. My eating habits were so bad that my physique was crazy looking the way I wanted her to look and I didn't care at all. I was eating McDonald's left and right. I eat Chinese buffets which I was called greasy foods and my native foods which always have greased, but very delicious. From time to time, I realize that I will tremendously struggle with my weight and also my transformation in my physique. I was working hard in the gym; the hard work was not showing because of the foods that I'm consuming every day. The symmetry was barely showing, the fat was covering my muscles and the definitions. One thing that really has gotten to me was my breathing. Every time I run, I realized that my breathing was getting thicker and it was hard for me to breathe. Even though I will run the miles I needed to run, but still, there was a huge struggle I will go through to finish my run and at the finishing point, my breathing will even get worse. Then I decided to change my whole diet and deciding to eat healthily. I start researching the healthy foods; ask my wife Vera who is vegan and definitely Mama Ruby who is always eating Healthy. When I began to start eating healthy, I mean everything has changed from worst to better. Even though my immune system has taken the time to get adjusted to my new healthy way of eating, but now I'm reaping what I sow. My body is in better condition and health has much improves since. Eating Healthy has also made my fatigue go away and I realized the foods I was consuming used to get me tired and now it seems to go away. I feel more energized since I been eating healthy. I'm more energetic, I work out longer and still have the strength to do whatever I want to do. Now I'm going to talk about the benefits of Eating Healthy. Eating Healthy can help you reduce the risks of heart disease by maintaining high blood pressure and also cholesterol levels. It can also help you control your weight. Another example of Eating Healthy is that it reduces your risks of chronic disease such as cancer, heart disease, and others... Eating Healthy leads to a pleasant lifestyle, beautiful attitude, positive attitude and something to look forward in the future. Eating Healthy makes you be in control of your health and life because of it just anything that you putting in your body. You have control of what goes in your body and know what it does to your body. You will only know what foods are good for your body by eating healthy. Perhaps I strongly believe eating healthy makes you feel better. It helps you mentally and spiritually. It is something that can't really be explained why that is, but you are more relaxed and think clearly. A study shows Fiber Foods, like complex carbohydrates, that contain soluble fiber can slow the absorption of sugar into your bloodstream and increase serotonin, the "feel good" chemical, both of which decrease mood swings. And the last thing before I go to the next topic, First thing in the morning before you put anything in your mouth, drink a glass of water. As I was online, I came across this government site which shows eight ways of Eating Healthy. The name of the site called HHS which stands for U.S. Department of Health & Human Services and according to this site those are the eight ways of Eating Healthy: Make half your plate fruits and vegetables: Choose red, orange, and dark-green vegetables like tomatoes, sweet potatoes, and broccoli, along with other vegetables for your meals. Add fruit to meals as part of main or side dishes or as dessert. The more colorful you make your plate, the more likely you are to get the vitamins, minerals, and fiber your body needs to be healthy. Make half the grains you eat whole grains: An easy way to eat more whole grains is to switch from a refined-grain food to a whole-grain food. For example, eat whole-wheat bread instead of white bread. Read the ingredients list and choose products that list whole-grain ingredients first. Look for things like: "whole wheat," "brown rice," "bulgur," "buckwheat," "oatmeal," "rolled oats," quinoa," or "wild rice." Switch to fat-free or low-fat (1%) milk: Both have the same amount of calcium and other essential nutrients as whole milk, but fewer calories and less saturated fat. Choose a variety of lean protein foods: Meat, poultry, seafood, dry beans or peas, eggs, nuts, and seeds are considered part of the protein foods group. Select leaner cuts of ground beef (where the label says 90% lean or higher), turkey breast, or chicken breast. Compare sodium in foods: Use the Nutrition Facts label to choose lower sodium versions of foods like soup, bread, and frozen meals. Select canned foods labeled "low sodium," "reduced sodium," or "no salt added." Drink water instead of sugary drinks: Cut calories by drinking water or unsweetened beverages. Soda, energy drinks, and sports drinks are a major source of added sugar and calories in American diets. Try adding a slice of lemon, lime, or watermelon or a splash of 100% juice to your glass of water if you want some flavor. Eat some seafood: Seafood includes fish (such as salmon, tuna, and trout) and shellfish (such as crab, mussels, and oysters). Seafood has protein, minerals, and omega-3 fatty acids (a heart-healthy fat). Adults should try to eat at least eight ounces a week of a variety of seafood. Children can eat smaller amounts of seafood, too. Cut back on solid fats: Eat fewer foods that contain solid fats. The major sources for Americans are cakes, cookies, and other desserts (often made with butter, margarine, or shortening); pizza; processed and fatty meats (e.g., sausages, hot dogs, bacon, ribs); and ice cream." It is very true. As a bodybuilder myself, I eat healthily and most of the foods mentioned are mostly what I also eat to sit fit and eat during my diet before a competition. The next topic will be talking about Dieting before Competition time.

 # DIETING

Dieting is very important when it comes to Bodybuilding. I hate Dieting; I hate it and hate it. Dieting plays a crucial role in your fitness life especially when you are competing against other competitors. Dieting is a final finishing touch to your masterpiece you been working for some time now, even months and years. This is what makes your physique looks phenomenal. Dieting is the main ingredient to your successful physique and attracts people to you when they see your physique on stage or wherever you go. This is what makes you stand out among others especially when your diet is on point. Dieting in the fitness is a league on his own which means that your Diet has to be on point at all times. I remembered the first time I tried to diet for my first show in Antelope Valley, I almost lost my mind. I taught it was going to be easy, but I was definitely wrong. I have to eat certain foods that I never ate before and were not what I ate as usual. My water intake has been measured and limited. I also have to watch everything that I eat and even drink. It was not fun at all because my coaches believe in the process, so I had to continue with the Dieting. Most of the foods that I was eating: Meat, almonds nuts, vegetables, brown rice, sweet potatoes, spinach, lots of fish, egg, oatmeal, fewer fruits because of the sugar intake, turkey breast, chicken breast, avocado, brown rice, whole grains, dried beans, and seeds. I have to stay away from any food that contains fat, sugar, and salt. Actually, when you look at my diet, it sucks because it's less tasty than an average person's food. It's not foods that an average person will prefer and eat because the food has no taste. My salt intake was limited and I will say almost everything. My diet was restricted diet and complicated. Everything that I was going to eat or eating, I have to make sure that it was not interfering with my diet. However, for the average person who is trying to diet and do the dieting stuff, he/she does not have to do the restricted diet. He/she still has to eat healthily, but not follow our restricted diet because we are bodybuilders and we intend to take the dieting thing a little extra notch. We are more focusing depriving ourselves those things that an average person won't do to their bodies and we do them. As for the average person, your job is to focus on losing weight or maintaining your weight whatever you feel that works for you. For you to get there, check out those eight foods that I listed in the previous topic Eating Healthy will help achieve your goals. As for us bodybuilders, we are more like artists. We are more focus on sculpting our bodies and with a restricted and perfect diet, the masterpiece comes to life. Instead of only focusing on one particular body parts, we are rounded when it comes to sculpting our bodies and that's how we do with our dieting. We try to balance everything because we are trying to create an amazing physique and something out of ordinary. Something that is never seen before and that will attract anyone that will glance at it. A crazy physique that will be the middle of attention, during our dieting, there are many rules that we have to follow the bodybuilders. For instance, we have to drink 1 to two gallon of water a day to flush all the toxins out of our bodies. We stop eating salt, oily foods; mostly eat lean and more foods that contain more proteins that will help keep our bodies lean, ripped and tight. As we get closer to competition's date, our diet gets more completed because we have to let certain foods go and keep eating certain over and over until the competition. The water intake has to diminish and instead of drinking two gallons of water, it goes down to one gallon and as it goes on the water intake keep dropping until the day before the competition, there is no water intake at all to keep the body dry and tight until show time. Now the next topic will talk about Competition.

 # COMPETITION

Competition is something that really excites me because of different various reasons. The first reason is when you meet your team again and you guys are back together. Secondly, it's when you meet other competitors that you haven't see for months and even a year and can't wait to hang out with them. Third, it's when you see new faces that are there to compete against you and even with you on the same stage, but it is so exciting to see them. Then as the list goes on, Competition overall is a great thing. You have different categories that eventually will be on the stage to show their packages. You perhaps guess to see different physique and when you taught you have seen it all, but I guess you are wrong. Those physiques that those competitors bring are really amazing and sometimes I strongly believe that the human body is a masterpiece. The human body is an artwork that really amazes me every time I see a different competitor with a whole new and different package on stage. During Competition, it's where I learn most about myself, my physique, what I really need to work on as a Bodybuilder and perhaps discovering my weaknesses. Now I know and have the ideas what I need to work on to be better for the next Competition. Competing against one another is also motivating me to be the best I can be. It brings out the greatness out of me and I don't intend to stop right now. I realize that during Competition time has been schooling time for me due to the fact I see something new also from the veterans of the sport. Every time I taught I saw it all, but I guess I was wrong. There was something new, different, bold, exciting, and great. As a Bodybuilder and athlete, I thought the veterans will retire and relaxed, but neither of one those because the veterans are even more hungry to show their better package on stage then the newcomers. Competition is divided into various categories and my category is Men's Open Bodybuilding. I can really list of the categories, but they are so many of them and it is a long list; so, if you want to look it up, please go on Musclemania.com site and you find them all. The next topic will be on the organization of Musclemania and Politics.

# MUSCLEMANIA AND POLITICS

Musclemania is the World's premier natural bodybuilding organization with physique fitness, sports model, and natural bodybuilding competitors. Musclemania is a huge organization and all over the world. As for me, I have been an athlete for this organization for the past 4 years now and I saw things that I need to be fixed and the politics that make competitors don't even want to be at this organization anymore. I won't speak for everybody, but I saw for myself and things that happened to me during that time why I was competing. Before I go into details, I want really show my appreciation for this organization and the support for the natural athletes who compete in this organization, but only give their full support to the athletes whom they like and feel they are beneficial to their organization. Musclemania intends to promote those athletes that they want to promote and seem to forget or I will say don't care about the remaining athletes who pay their hard-earned money to compete for them, but Musclemania will tell you that they are fair and firm which I hardly believe it is true. I'm an athlete, published author, father of four, student and also a businessman; so, everything that I do, it has been or it is calculated already before my involvement. Joining

Musclemania is a life learning experience on my part. I had learned a lot of things while competing and presently still do. My patience has increased while competing and I mean by that, there were times when I competed against other competitors, the crowd went crazy and feel good to give a great show. There were times when I went against competitors who I strongly think that should not have won, but still, they give it to them for whatever reasons. Even the crowd was not pleased to the judges' calls and really talking about the whole situation. There were times that I should have taken first place, but my spot was given to another athlete because the owner of the organization has called the wrong name, but is okay, that is life and life goes on. There were times, Musclemania wouldn't play the song for my posing routine, but rather played house music that didn't go with my routine pose at all. The last one that I really make me laugh was the last show I did in Burbank, California in 2018 in October. My physique was solid and everything else was on point, but still gives it to someone else which I wasn't surprised at all. Usually, it will get to me, but I just figurate it out that I'm not competing because of them, but for myself because it makes me happy and I love competing. This is what most of the athletes go through all the times and that's not fair at all. This is how I feel, if I lose, let me lose to someone who is better than me and whom I can learn from, but not a person who looks up to me and suddenly he wins but doesn't even know that he won and looks as surprised as everyone else including the crowd. As I speak right now, I don't care about any trophies neither prices. I do it for the love of the sport, not for Musclemania or anyone else without disrespecting anyone. If Musclemania wants to do the right thing, they will do so. Who am I to tell them how to run their business because before I got there was a Musclemania already and if I leave they will still be there. As for me, integrity is everything to me and it's up to them to do what is right. Even though politics and unfairness are evidence to most of the competitors not succeeding in their crafts; but the Networking that Musclemania brings is undeniable and its evidence why she is one of the biggest natural bodybuilding organization in the world.

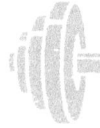

# THE NETWORKING

Networking is fun and everything. Networking is when a person links with another person for the purpose of their resources, best interests of each other, what they can offer each other, bring to the table or process of interacting with others to exchange information and develop professional or social contacts. Networking is how most of the bodybuilders make their money and living because the organization itself is not paying them enough, but gives them the exposure they are looking for as athletes. For instance, for me, I exchange my cell number, email, social media info with different and various athletes I feel that we have something in common. Sometimes it is the opposite, other athletes see me and they admire my workout ethics and want to do something that will both benefit us and give more exposure by opening more venues. One thing I love about Networking is that you get to meet new faces, new people and all over the world. You get to know them and where they are from. You also get to hang out with them for a couple days and share information just in case one day you go compete to the venue and perhaps at least you know someone there already that make it easy for you to get around. Throughout Networking I get to build solid friendships with people that I never taught I wouldn't have with.

Perhaps I get to have a connection and place to stay just in case if I'm competing in their location and save me money instead of paying for a hotel. Through Networking, a fitness friend can hook you up with a gig. For example, most of the fitness competitors also do modeling, some of them like me are inspiring actors, models, fitness models, published authors and even know agencies that can help another fitness athlete to make their dream comes true. Networking does open lots of avenues, opportunities for fitness athletes and which can to traveling and even traveling in the future.

# TRAVELING

Since I been competing as a Natural Bodybuilding, I have been also traveling a lot. I have been locally traveling back and forth. I had competed in Lancaster in the Antelope Valley, Burbank, California, and San Diego if I'm not mistaken but I'm not so sure because it was during my first show. I also had competed out of California. I had competed in Las Vegas at Golden Nuggets. I had also competed in South Miami, Beach, and Florida at the Colony Theater. Perhaps only that I had competed locally, but also traveled internationally to be one of the judges in Japan, an island name Saipan. I was a great experience and I'm grateful for Grady gray who has taken me under his wings in this Bodybuilding world and still doing great things for me. Before we head to Saipan, I stopped in Okinawa where Grady and his family stays. Okinawa is one of the most beautiful places I've ever been and I fell in love with it when I visited. People of Okinawa are very genuine, caring, respectful and very kind toward the tourists. Lot of Americans do live there and also it is a beautiful island. Any way when Grady and I, we traveled to Saipan to become judges and guess posers the Saipan at Dee Clayton Classic Show, it was an experience that I couldn't forget and people there gave us this warmed welcome which made feel like a home again. I also thank Grady and Dee Clayton for the opportunity that they both gave me and forever grateful for that. It was once in a lifetime experience to go somewhere where you have no clue how things are going to turn out, but turned out beautifully, admiration and respect that Grady and I, we both received from the competitors and people of Saipan. Grady and I, we put in a 5 stars hotels and so of everything else were also provided for us. We stayed there for a couple of days, traveled to other islands, visited a cave and other places that were very adventurous to visit. Those are one of the places where you visit and don't want to come back. It's peaceful and I love it. Grady and I received awards for being judges and guess posers. The welcome was warmed and great. We enjoyed ourselves and even went out with some of the competitors to celebrate in the night. On our way coming back to Okinawa, if not mistaken, it was a typhoon, so we have to stay at one Grady's friend house in Guam which is another beautiful place in Japan, but barely had a glance at it. Just recently which was last year, Vera, my soul mate and I, we traveled to Okinawa to go visit Grady and his family and I had a show there also in Tokyo in Shibuya. Grady and I, we did an NPCJ show with the rest of the GrayAtlas athletes. It was another great experience to have. A few days later, after the show, when Grady and I, we returned back to Okinawa to meet our family, It just hit me when I was alone upstairs in the room by myself. Fitness is part of me and something that I really enjoy doing and which leads to my next topic.

# FITNESS IS A LIFESTYLE

Fitness is a lifestyle for me. I enjoy it and love doing it. Again I'm 36 years old and I look like I'm in my early 20s. I love when people guess my age and when I tell them how old I am, see them fill with surprise on their faces. Fitness has changed my life completely and that's the naked truth. Not only that, it has brought me joy, but also a fitness family that will forever be part of me till my dying day. Fitness has made me a better person. Besides praying, I use fitness to meditate and fight my demons. I will explain what I meant by that, whenever something is bothering or angry at someone and I know I'm about to lose control, I go to the gym ASAP and release all the frustrations on the weights. When I'm done working out, I feel like a brand new person, I'm calmer, relax, thinking clearly and most importantly not angry anymore and that's a good reliever. Through my fitness journey, I have touched the souls of ordinary people just like me, met great people, met interesting people, and met some of my favorite bodybuilders local and international. Fitness has put me in a great space where I'm able to reach and help people all over the world. For example, look at social media, while working out I will download a workout video on Instagram, Facebook and snapshot. People go crazy over it and that alone that's what makes me keep on doing what I'm doing, my friend. It is very rewarding not as money wise, but mostly as touching souls and inspiring people around the world and the seven continents. That's what I want and love doing. Fitness has turned me from a skinny kid who barely has any muscle to someone who now is muscular as a superhero. Fitness has made me appreciate my health lot more, gave me more confidence and I am so blessed for that. I have been through a lot since I was born. I was a premature baby and I barely made it, but God has refused to let me go. I used to weigh 120 pounds when I was in my early twenties, but now I'm 192 pounds. 2012 ending of that year, my life was almost cut short right before my own eyes. I hit my head on a construction crank while working for Inter-con Security Company. The doctor has to give me seven stitches all because of trying to be a great father to my children. Not only that I survived because of God's love but also because of Fitness. I always kept myself in great shape. I work out five days a week doing a different variation of exercises. In the same year, my head injury has continuously given me several migraines every other day. I would bleed from time to time in my right nasal. Fitness has kept me going and kept me strong as years come. My right knee has been dislocated and through Fitness I find a way to heal the pain. When I take my shirt off, when you look closely, you realize my back is uneven because I broke it. In 1998 on the Buduburam Camp in Ghana which is the refugee camp, while playing soccer, I don't remember exactly what happened, but the next day I couldn't walk, sleep and lay down, stand and even sit. The pain was so severe that I could do was to cry. The pain went on for months and months until one of my uncles has used some herbals and every morning and everything he would walk on my back by massaging it to put it back together. Before our departure, my back was getting better and some. In February, we arrived in the United States and I made a decision that will completely change my whole entire life. I decided not to be the victim of this back injury that I have. I decided working out by only using my own body weight and with twenty five pounds dumbbells for about four years. I built up strength that I never had before by doing a thousand pushups in different variation and sit-ups also which helped to strengthen my back muscles. My physique has also changed tremendously in a good way. For me, Fitness has been part of me for so long. I will say about 20 years now since I been working out and still learning something every day in this Fitness world. It is part of me and it's like a marriage. I will be faithful to her until I leave this world. For anyone who is trying to get into Fitness, don't hesitate and go for it because it will be the greatest investment you have done in your life. It's rewarding and you will benefit every piece of it. If I can do it, which means you can do it also.

    First I want to thank God for making everything possible for my family. I want to take the time to give a special thanks to my soulmate Vera who has always been by my side from day one and has my better half since. I also to thank Liam Sean from Urlink Print&Media for giving a lifetime opportunity and making it possible for this book to see the light. I want to thank the whole Urlink Print&Media staffs for their hard work. I want to thank Grady Gray who has the vision for me becoming a Bodybuilder, Osei Bonsu who never hesitated to show me his secrets how to build a crazy physique, Brother Duke giving me tips on the legs workout, Raquel who always tells me the raw truth and that alone motivates me more. I also want to take the time and say thank to my brothers: McKees and Nelson who always bring out the best of me when working out. I want to thank the whole Team California, GrayAtlas &Atlasphysique Family for been there for me since day one. I really appreciate you guys always. I also want to thank my mentor, our mom, the one and only Ruby Carter Pikes for everything and life period. I really mean it from the bottom of my heart. Thank you to all my supporters and for making this book becoming a bestseller. Other special thanks to Samson B Toe who always persuaded me to write a fitness book and Joelter G Toe who have always been there for me and my children.

Check the clothing brand the author modeled https://www.grayatlasfit.com/
Author was also featured in the movie Art of Deception by Richard Ryan (https://www.imdb.me/RichardRyan. More information here http://www.oxfilms.us/

Social media pages:
Instagram:@prcmember80
Facebook:@princetoesr
Snapchat:@PRC Member

www.ingramcontent.com/pod-product-compliance
Ingram Content Group UK Ltd.
Pitfield, Milton Keynes, MK11 3LW, UK
UKHW022219230426
12048UKWH00016BA/952